Personal Trainer Student Log Book

by
William Murrell

Bloomington, IN

Milton Keynes, UK

AuthorHouse™
1663 Liberty Drive, Suite 200
Bloomington, IN 47403
www.authorhouse.com
Phone: 1-800-839-8640

AuthorHouse™ UK Ltd.
500 Avebury Boulevard
Central Milton Keynes, MK9 2BE
www.authorhouse.co.uk
Phone: 08001974150

First published by AuthorHouse 5/18/2006

ISBN: 1-4259-2438-7 (sc)

Printed in the United States of America
Bloomington, Indiana

This book is printed on acid-free paper.

Strongly Advised.

This program is not a cure or an aide to counter act any medical recommendations. Before using this program it is strongly suggested that you seek or visit a physician if you have any medical problems or handicaps.

Introduction

One question a lot of people would like to know is how you introduce yourself to a new change. Is it basic will power, determination, desire, or just mind over matter? The answer is, all the above and this booklet is designed to encourage those among anything else to initiate the power of determination and to show you how to develop. It is to take you from your current basic or intermediate understanding to an elevated enterprise of working out. This guided documentation is to help introduce you to the concept and designed patterns associated with the human anatomy and to allow you to chronicalize your achievements over a period of time, giving you a broader perspective than you would get from a day-to-day memory. The book can be used as a yardstick by which to measure your performance in the gym or life thus pointing out the paths of strengths and weaknesses. Life as we see it now is a fast pace foot race, but rather it should be a happy and healthy journey to well being. A healthy body is everything now. If need be, take a look over your left shoulder at the competition of fit models, movie stars, gym hunks, swimsuit models and give yourself that extra push towards excellence. The examples of those who met untimely ends because the body didn't matter remind us that the finish line can be anywhere. There is no deadline quite like death, so you may as well go ahead and become a healthy and fit person while you still can. Take care of your body. You are the only one who can.

Important:

Personal trainers have to be mindful that all students are not built the same nor have the same endurance. The process as you know through experience will be gradual but you also have to take notice if the student is putting forth the necessary effort to reaching a new goal. Sometime it may be necessary to push the student a little because of the lack of motivation or attentiveness. Be sure you continue to follow necessary protocol of doing a health assessment before doing any workout routine with the student to prevent any litigation or arraignment.

Daily Fitness Assessment

Upper and Lower Body Workout Routines

Chest	Back	Biceps
1. Barbell Bench Press	1. Seated Cable Row	1. Alternating Cable Curls
2. Barbell Incline Press	2. Wide Grip Lat Pulldowns	2. Seated Concentration Curls
3. Dumbbell Incline Press	3. Front V-Bar Pulldowns	3. Hammer Curls
4. Cable Crossover	4. Low Row Extensions	4. Standing EZ Curls
5. Flyes / Pectorials	5. Straight Bar Standing Pulldowns	5. Dumbbell Curls
6. Dumbbell Bench Press	6. Hi-Ro Extensions	6. Barbell Curls
7. Dumbell Flys	7. Dumbbell Rows	
8. Pullovers	8. T- Bar Rows	
9. Dumbbell Incline Pec Press		

Shoulders	Biceps	Triceps
1. Seated Military Presses	1. Alternating Cable Curls	1. Seated Tricep Presses
2. Front Cable Raises	2. Seated Concentration Curls	2. Triceps Kickbacks
3. Side Dumbell Lateral Raises	3. Hammer Curls	3. Triceps Pushdowns
4. Reverse Flyes	4. Standing EZ Curls	4. Bench Dips
5. Dumbbell Front Raises	5. Dumbbell Curls	5. Alternating Standing Extensions
6. Barbell Upright Rows	6. Barbell Curls	6. Reverse Tricep Presses
7. Side Cable Lateral Raises		7. Overhead Bumbell Extensions
Trapsezius		
1. Standing Front Barbell Rows		

Quadriceps	Hamstrings	Abdominals
1. Barbell Squats	1. Dumbbell Lunges	1. Flat Bench Leg Raises
2. Leg Presses	2. Lying Leg Curls	2. Bent Knee Raises
3. Leg Extensions	3. Staight-Leg Deadlifts	3. Machine Crunches
4. Hack Squats	4. Standing Leg Curls	4. Lying Twisting Crunches
5. Lunges	**Calves**	5. Seated Twisting Crunches
	1. Seated Calf Raises	6. Single Plate Twisting Crunches
	2. Standing Heel Raises	
	3. Donkey Calf Raises	
	4. One Leg Calf Raises	

Diagram of Fitness Chart

Routine Exercise Chart

Week ________________ **Date** ________________

Exercise - Biceps

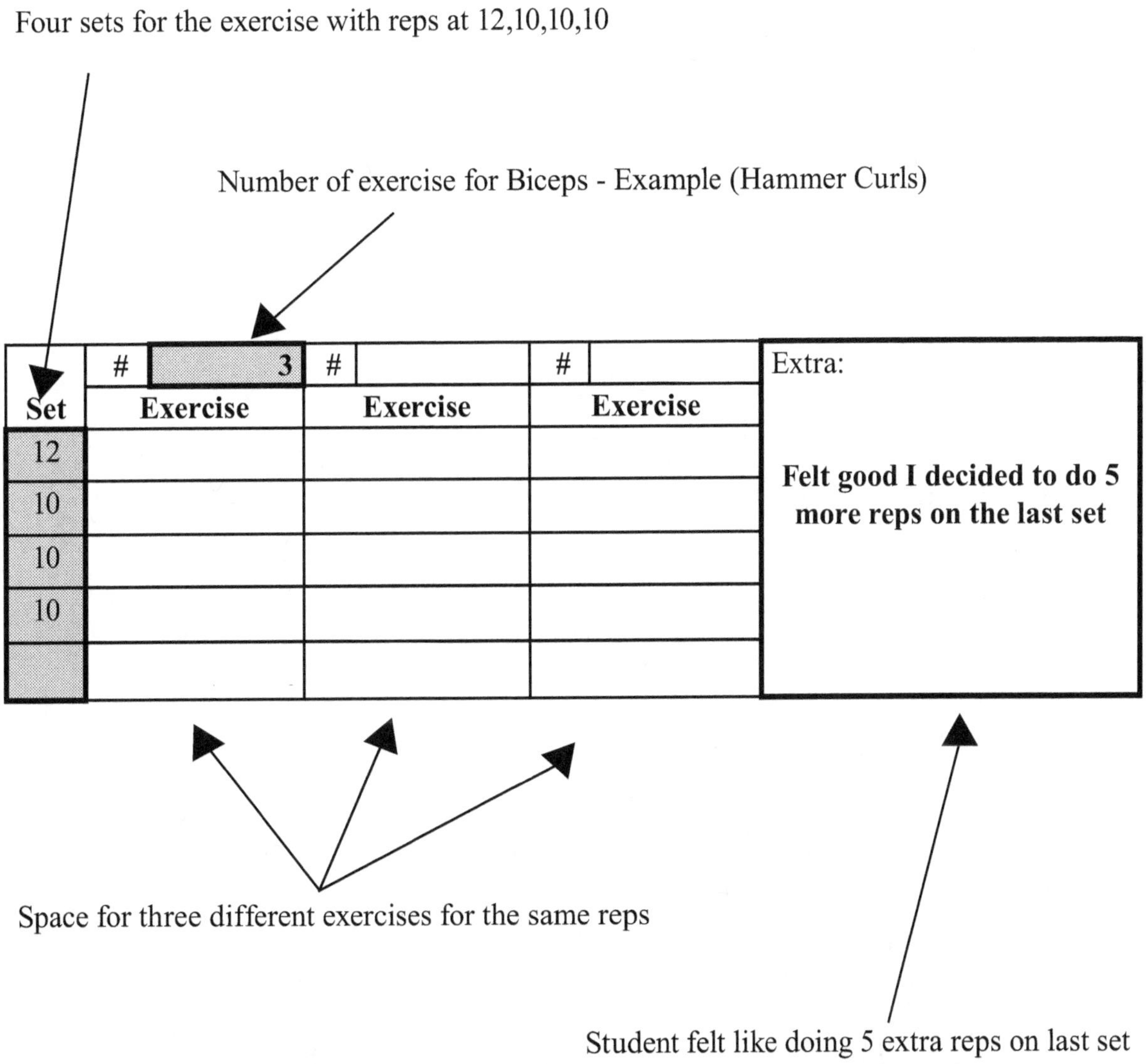

Four sets for the exercise with reps at 12,10,10,10

Number of exercise for Biceps - Example (Hammer Curls)

Set	# 3 Exercise	# Exercise	# Exercise	Extra:
12				**Felt good I decided to do 5 more reps on the last set**
10				
10				
10				

Space for three different exercises for the same reps

Student felt like doing 5 extra reps on last set

Student Information

STUDENT 1

Student Name ______________________________

Address ______________________________

____

Phone (cell) ______________________________

(home) ______________________________

Email ______________________________

Goals:

1.________________________
2.________________________
3.________________________
4.________________________
5.________________________
6.________________________
7.________________________
8.________________________

Body Measurements

Before		After	
Body Fat _____	Neck ______	Body Fat _____	Neck ______
Chest _____	Waist ______	Chest _____	Waist ______
Hips _____		Hips _____	

Weight _______

Weight _______

Daily Fitness Assessment

STUDENT 1

Routine Exercise Chart

Week ________________ Date ______________

Exercise _____________

Set	#	#	#	Extra:
	Exercise	**Exercise**	**Exercise**	

Exercise _____________

Set	#	#	#	Extra:
	Exercise	**Exercise**	**Exercise**	

Exercise _____________

Set	#	#	#	Extra:
	Exercise	**Exercise**	**Exercise**	

Exercise _____________

Set	#	#	#	Extra:
	Exercise	**Exercise**	**Exercise**	

Exercise _____________

Set	#	#	#	Extra:
	Exercise	**Exercise**	**Exercise**	

Exercise _____________

Set	#	#	#	Extra:
	Exercise	**Exercise**	**Exercise**	

Brief notes for student

STUDENT 1

Daily Fitness Assessment

Routine Exercise Chart

Week ________________ **Date** ________________

Exercise _____________

Set	# Exercise	# Exercise	# Exercise	Extra:

Exercise _____________

Set	# Exercise	# Exercise	# Exercise	Extra:

Exercise _____________

Set	# Exercise	# Exercise	# Exercise	Extra:

Exercise _____________

Set	# Exercise	# Exercise	# Exercise	Extra:

Exercise _____________

Set	# Exercise	# Exercise	# Exercise	Extra:

Exercise _____________

Set	# Exercise	# Exercise	# Exercise	Extra:

Brief notes for student

STUDENT 1

Daily Fitness Assessment

Routine Exercise Chart

Week ________________ **Date** ________________

Exercise _____________

Set	#	#	#	Extra:
	Exercise	**Exercise**	**Exercise**	

Exercise _____________

Set	#	#	#	Extra:
	Exercise	**Exercise**	**Exercise**	

Exercise _____________

Set	#	#	#	Extra:
	Exercise	**Exercise**	**Exercise**	

Exercise _____________

Set	#	#	#	Extra:
	Exercise	**Exercise**	**Exercise**	

Exercise _____________

Set	#	#	#	Extra:
	Exercise	**Exercise**	**Exercise**	

Exercise _____________

Set	#	#	#	Extra:
	Exercise	**Exercise**	**Exercise**	

Brief notes for student

STUDENT 1

Daily Fitness Assessment

Routine Exercise Chart

Week ________________ **Date** ________________

Exercise ______________

	#	#	#	Extra:
Set	**Exercise**	**Exercise**	**Exercise**	

Exercise ______________

	#	#	#	Extra:
Set	**Exercise**	**Exercise**	**Exercise**	

Exercise ______________

	#	#	#	Extra:
Set	**Exercise**	**Exercise**	**Exercise**	

Exercise ______________

	#	#	#	Extra:
Set	**Exercise**	**Exercise**	**Exercise**	

Exercise ______________

	#	#	#	Extra:
Set	**Exercise**	**Exercise**	**Exercise**	

Exercise ______________

	#	#	#	Extra:
Set	**Exercise**	**Exercise**	**Exercise**	

Brief notes for student

Daily Fitness Assessment

STUDENT 1

Routine Exercise Chart

Week ________________ **Date** ________________

Exercise _____________

Set	#		#		#		Extra:
	Exercise		**Exercise**		**Exercise**		

Exercise _____________

Set	#		#		#		Extra:
	Exercise		**Exercise**		**Exercise**		

Exercise _____________

Set	#		#		#		Extra:
	Exercise		**Exercise**		**Exercise**		

Exercise _____________

Set	#		#		#		Extra:
	Exercise		**Exercise**		**Exercise**		

Exercise _____________

Set	#		#		#		Extra:
	Exercise		**Exercise**		**Exercise**		

Exercise _____________

Set	#		#		#		Extra:
	Exercise		**Exercise**		**Exercise**		

Brief notes for student

STUDENT 1

Daily Fitness Assessment

Routine Exercise Chart

Week ________________ **Date** _______________

Exercise _____________

Set	#	#	#	Extra:
	Exercise	**Exercise**	**Exercise**	

Exercise _____________

Set	#	#	#	Extra:
	Exercise	**Exercise**	**Exercise**	

Exercise _____________

Set	#	#	#	Extra:
	Exercise	**Exercise**	**Exercise**	

Exercise _____________

Set	#	#	#	Extra:
	Exercise	**Exercise**	**Exercise**	

Exercise _____________

Set	#	#	#	Extra:
	Exercise	**Exercise**	**Exercise**	

Exercise _____________

Set	#	#	#	Extra:
	Exercise	**Exercise**	**Exercise**	

Brief notes for student

Daily Fitness Assessment

STUDENT 1

Routine Exercise Chart

Week ________________ **Date** _______________

Exercise _____________

Set	#		#		#		Extra:
	Exercise		**Exercise**		**Exercise**		

Exercise _____________

Set	#		#		#		Extra:
	Exercise		**Exercise**		**Exercise**		

Exercise _____________

Set	#		#		#		Extra:
	Exercise		**Exercise**		**Exercise**		

Exercise _____________

Set	#		#		#		Extra:
	Exercise		**Exercise**		**Exercise**		

Exercise _____________

Set	#		#		#		Extra:
	Exercise		**Exercise**		**Exercise**		

Exercise _____________

Set	#		#		#		Extra:
	Exercise		**Exercise**		**Exercise**		

Brief notes for student

STUDENT 1

Daily Fitness Assessment

Routine Exercise Chart

Week ________________ **Date** ________________

Exercise _____________

Set	#		#		#		Extra:
	Exercise		**Exercise**		**Exercise**		

Exercise _____________

Set	#		#		#		Extra:
	Exercise		**Exercise**		**Exercise**		

Exercise _____________

Set	#		#		#		Extra:
	Exercise		**Exercise**		**Exercise**		

Exercise _____________

Set	#		#		#		Extra:
	Exercise		**Exercise**		**Exercise**		

Exercise _____________

Set	#		#		#		Extra:
	Exercise		**Exercise**		**Exercise**		

Exercise _____________

Set	#		#		#		Extra:
	Exercise		**Exercise**		**Exercise**		

Brief notes for student

Daily Fitness Assessment

STUDENT 1

Routine Exercise Chart

Week ________________ Date ______________

Exercise _____________

Set	#		#		#		Extra:
	Exercise		**Exercise**		**Exercise**		

Exercise _____________

Set	#		#		#		Extra:
	Exercise		**Exercise**		**Exercise**		

Exercise _____________

Set	#		#		#		Extra:
	Exercise		**Exercise**		**Exercise**		

Exercise _____________

Set	#		#		#		Extra:
	Exercise		**Exercise**		**Exercise**		

Exercise _____________

Set	#		#		#		Extra:
	Exercise		**Exercise**		**Exercise**		

Exercise _____________

Set	#		#		#		Extra:
	Exercise		**Exercise**		**Exercise**		

Brief notes for student

Daily Fitness Assessment

STUDENT 1

Routine Exercise Chart

Week ________________ Date ________________

Exercise _____________

Set	#		#		#		Extra:
	Exercise		Exercise		Exercise		

Exercise _____________

Set	#		#		#		Extra:
	Exercise		Exercise		Exercise		

Exercise _____________

Set	#		#		#		Extra:
	Exercise		Exercise		Exercise		

Exercise _____________

Set	#		#		#		Extra:
	Exercise		Exercise		Exercise		

Exercise _____________

Set	#		#		#		Extra:
	Exercise		Exercise		Exercise		

Exercise _____________

Set	#		#		#		Extra:
	Exercise		Exercise		Exercise		

Brief notes for student

STUDENT 1

Daily Fitness Assessment

Routine Exercise Chart

Week ________________ **Date** _______________

Exercise _____________

Set	#		#		#		Extra:
	Exercise		**Exercise**		**Exercise**		

Exercise _____________

Set	#		#		#		Extra:
	Exercise		**Exercise**		**Exercise**		

Exercise _____________

Set	#		#		#		Extra:
	Exercise		**Exercise**		**Exercise**		

Exercise _____________

Set	#		#		#		Extra:
	Exercise		**Exercise**		**Exercise**		

Exercise _____________

Set	#		#		#		Extra:
	Exercise		**Exercise**		**Exercise**		

Exercise _____________

Set	#		#		#		Extra:
	Exercise		**Exercise**		**Exercise**		

Brief notes for student

STUDENT 1

Daily Fitness Assessment

Routine Exercise Chart

Week ________________ **Date** _______________

Exercise _____________

Set	#		#		#		Extra:
	Exercise		**Exercise**		**Exercise**		

Exercise _____________

Set	#		#		#		Extra:
	Exercise		**Exercise**		**Exercise**		

Exercise _____________

Set	#		#		#		Extra:
	Exercise		**Exercise**		**Exercise**		

Exercise _____________

Set	#		#		#		Extra:
	Exercise		**Exercise**		**Exercise**		

Exercise _____________

Set	#		#		#		Extra:
	Exercise		**Exercise**		**Exercise**		

Exercise _____________

Set	#		#		#		Extra:
	Exercise		**Exercise**		**Exercise**		

Brief notes for student

Daily Fitness Assessment

Routine Exercise Chart

Week ______________ Date ______________

Exercise ____________

Set	#		#		#		Extra:
	Exercise		Exercise		Exercise		

Exercise ____________

Set	#		#		#		Extra:
	Exercise		Exercise		Exercise		

Exercise ____________

Set	#		#		#		Extra:
	Exercise		Exercise		Exercise		

Exercise ____________

Set	#		#		#		Extra:
	Exercise		Exercise		Exercise		

Exercise ____________

Set	#		#		#		Extra:
	Exercise		Exercise		Exercise		

Exercise ____________

Set	#		#		#		Extra:
	Exercise		Exercise		Exercise		

Brief notes for student

Daily Fitness Assessment

STUDENT 1

Routine Exercise Chart

Week ________________ **Date** _______________

Exercise _____________

Set	#		#		#		Extra:
	Exercise		**Exercise**		**Exercise**		

Exercise _____________

Set	#		#		#		Extra:
	Exercise		**Exercise**		**Exercise**		

Exercise _____________

Set	#		#		#		Extra:
	Exercise		**Exercise**		**Exercise**		

Exercise _____________

Set	#		#		#		Extra:
	Exercise		**Exercise**		**Exercise**		

Exercise _____________

Set	#		#		#		Extra:
	Exercise		**Exercise**		**Exercise**		

Exercise _____________

Set	#		#		#		Extra:
	Exercise		**Exercise**		**Exercise**		

Brief notes for student

Daily Fitness Assessment

STUDENT 1

Routine Exercise Chart

Week ________________ Date _______________

Exercise _____________

Set	#		#		#		Extra:
	Exercise		**Exercise**		**Exercise**		

Exercise _____________

Set	#		#		#		Extra:
	Exercise		**Exercise**		**Exercise**		

Exercise _____________

Set	#		#		#		Extra:
	Exercise		**Exercise**		**Exercise**		

Exercise _____________

Set	#		#		#		Extra:
	Exercise		**Exercise**		**Exercise**		

Exercise _____________

Set	#		#		#		Extra:
	Exercise		**Exercise**		**Exercise**		

Exercise _____________

Set	#		#		#		Extra:
	Exercise		**Exercise**		**Exercise**		

Brief notes for student

Daily Fitness Assessment

STUDENT 1

Total Body Workout

Cardio	Date ________		Date ________		Date ________	
	#		#		#	
		Time		Time		Time
1. Stationary Bike						
2. Treadmill						
3. Aerobic classes						
4. Racquetball						
5. Jump rope						
6. Ski machine						
7. Jogging						
8. Jumping jacks						
9. Boxing						
10. Basketball						
11. Walking						
12. Stair stepper						
13. Swimming						
14. Volleyball						
15. Water polo						
16. Rock climbing	Notes:		Notes:		Notes:	
17. Football						

Daily Fitness Assessment

STUDENT 1

Total Body Workout

	Date ________		Date ________		Date ________	
	#		#		#	
Cardio		**Time**		**Time**		**Time**
1. Stationary Bike						
2. Treadmill						
3. Aerobic classes						
4. Racquetball						
5. Jump rope						
6. Ski machine						
7. Jogging						
8. Jumping jacks						
9. Boxing						
10. Basketball						
11. Walking						
12. Stair stepper						
13. Swimming						
14. Volleyball						
15. Water polo						
16. Rock climbing	Notes:		Notes:		Notes:	
17. Football						

Daily Fitness Assessment

STUDENT 1

Total Body Workout

Cardio	Date ________		Date ________		Date ________	
	#		#		#	
		Time		Time		Time
1. Stationary Bike						
2. Treadmill						
3. Aerobic classes						
4. Racquetball						
5. Jump rope						
6. Ski machine						
7. Jogging						
8. Jumping jacks						
9. Boxing						
10. Basketball						
11. Walking						
12. Stair stepper						
13. Swimming						
14. Volleyball						
15. Water polo						
16. Rock climbing	Notes:		Notes:		Notes:	
17. Football						

Daily Fitness Assessment

STUDENT 1

Total Body Workout

	Date ________		Date ________		Date ________	
Cardio	#	**Time**	#	**Time**	#	**Time**
1. Stationary Bike						
2. Treadmill						
3. Aerobic classes						
4. Racquetball						
5. Jump rope						
6. Ski machine						
7. Jogging						
8. Jumping jacks						
9. Boxing						
10. Basketball						
11. Walking						
12. Stair stepper						
13. Swimming						
14. Volleyball						
15. Water polo						
16. Rock climbing	Notes:		Notes:		Notes:	
17. Football						

Daily Fitness Assessment

STUDENT 1

Total Body Workout

Date ________ Date ________ Date ________

Cardio	#		#		#	
	Time		Time		Time	
1. Stationary Bike						
2. Treadmill						
3. Aerobic classes						
4. Racquetball						
5. Jump rope						
6. Ski machine						
7. Jogging						
8. Jumping jacks						
9. Boxing						
10. Basketball						
11. Walking						
12. Stair stepper						
13. Swimming						
14. Volleyball						
15. Water polo						
16. Rock climbing	Notes:		Notes:		Notes:	
17. Football						

Student Information

Student Name ______________________________

Address ______________________________

____

Phone (cell) ______________________________

(home) ______________________________

Email ______________________________

Goals:

1.________________________
2.________________________
3.________________________
4.________________________
5.________________________
6.________________________
7.________________________
8.________________________

Body Measurements

Before

Body Fat _____ Neck ______
Chest _____ Waist ______
Hips _____

Weight _______

After

Body Fat _____ Neck ______
Chest _____ Waist ______
Hips _____

Weight _______

STUDENT 2

Daily Fitness Assessment

STUDENT 2

Routine Exercise Chart

Week ________________ **Date** _______________

Exercise _____________

Set	# Exercise	# Exercise	# Exercise	Extra:

Exercise _____________

Set	# Exercise	# Exercise	# Exercise	Extra:

Exercise _____________

Set	# Exercise	# Exercise	# Exercise	Extra:

Exercise _____________

Set	# Exercise	# Exercise	# Exercise	Extra:

Exercise _____________

Set	# Exercise	# Exercise	# Exercise	Extra:

Exercise _____________

Set	# Exercise	# Exercise	# Exercise	Extra:

Brief notes for student

Daily Fitness Assessment

STUDENT 2

Routine Exercise Chart

Week ________________ **Date** _______________

Exercise _____________

Set	#	#	#	Extra:
	Exercise	**Exercise**	**Exercise**	

Exercise _____________

Set	#	#	#	Extra:
	Exercise	**Exercise**	**Exercise**	

Exercise _____________

Set	#	#	#	Extra:
	Exercise	**Exercise**	**Exercise**	

Exercise _____________

Set	#	#	#	Extra:
	Exercise	**Exercise**	**Exercise**	

Exercise _____________

Set	#	#	#	Extra:
	Exercise	**Exercise**	**Exercise**	

Exercise _____________

Set	#	#	#	Extra:
	Exercise	**Exercise**	**Exercise**	

Brief notes for student

Daily Fitness Assessment

STUDENT 2

Routine Exercise Chart

Week _______________ **Date** _______________

Exercise ____________

Set	#		#		#		Extra:
	Exercise		**Exercise**		**Exercise**		

Exercise ____________

Set	#		#		#		Extra:
	Exercise		**Exercise**		**Exercise**		

Exercise ____________

Set	#		#		#		Extra:
	Exercise		**Exercise**		**Exercise**		

Exercise ____________

Set	#		#		#		Extra:
	Exercise		**Exercise**		**Exercise**		

Exercise ____________

Set	#		#		#		Extra:
	Exercise		**Exercise**		**Exercise**		

Exercise ____________

Set	#		#		#		Extra:
	Exercise		**Exercise**		**Exercise**		

Brief notes for student

Daily Fitness Assessment

STUDENT 2

Routine Exercise Chart

Week ________________ **Date** _______________

Exercise _____________

Set	# Exercise	# Exercise	# Exercise	Extra:

Exercise _____________

Set	# Exercise	# Exercise	# Exercise	Extra:

Exercise _____________

Set	# Exercise	# Exercise	# Exercise	Extra:

Exercise _____________

Set	# Exercise	# Exercise	# Exercise	Extra:

Exercise _____________

Set	# Exercise	# Exercise	# Exercise	Extra:

Exercise _____________

Set	# Exercise	# Exercise	# Exercise	Extra:

Brief notes for student

Daily Fitness Assessment

STUDENT 2

Routine Exercise Chart

Week _______________ **Date** ______________

Exercise ____________

Set	#		#		#		Extra:
	Exercise		**Exercise**		**Exercise**		

Exercise ____________

Set	#		#		#		Extra:
	Exercise		**Exercise**		**Exercise**		

Exercise ____________

Set	#		#		#		Extra:
	Exercise		**Exercise**		**Exercise**		

Exercise ____________

Set	#		#		#		Extra:
	Exercise		**Exercise**		**Exercise**		

Exercise ____________

Set	#		#		#		Extra:
	Exercise		**Exercise**		**Exercise**		

Exercise ____________

Set	#		#		#		Extra:
	Exercise		**Exercise**		**Exercise**		

Brief notes for student

Daily Fitness Assessment

STUDENT 2

Routine Exercise Chart

Week ________________ Date _______________

Exercise _____________

Set	#		#		#		Extra:
	Exercise		**Exercise**		**Exercise**		

Exercise _____________

Set	#		#		#		Extra:
	Exercise		**Exercise**		**Exercise**		

Exercise _____________

Set	#		#		#		Extra:
	Exercise		**Exercise**		**Exercise**		

Exercise _____________

Set	#		#		#		Extra:
	Exercise		**Exercise**		**Exercise**		

Exercise _____________

Set	#		#		#		Extra:
	Exercise		**Exercise**		**Exercise**		

Exercise _____________

Set	#		#		#		Extra:
	Exercise		**Exercise**		**Exercise**		

Brief notes for student

Daily Fitness Assessment

Routine Exercise Chart

Week ______________ **Date** ______________

Exercise ____________

Set	# Exercise	# Exercise	# Exercise	Extra:

Exercise ____________

Set	# Exercise	# Exercise	# Exercise	Extra:

STUDENT 2

Exercise ____________

Set	# Exercise	# Exercise	# Exercise	Extra:

Exercise ____________

Set	# Exercise	# Exercise	# Exercise	Extra:

Exercise ____________

Set	# Exercise	# Exercise	# Exercise	Extra:

Exercise ____________

Set	# Exercise	# Exercise	# Exercise	Extra:

Brief notes for student

Daily Fitness Assessment

Routine Exercise Chart

Week ________________ **Date** _______________

STUDENT 2

Exercise _____________

Set	#		#		#		Extra:
	Exercise		**Exercise**		**Exercise**		

Exercise _____________

Set	#		#		#		Extra:
	Exercise		**Exercise**		**Exercise**		

Exercise _____________

Set	#		#		#		Extra:
	Exercise		**Exercise**		**Exercise**		

Exercise _____________

Set	#		#		#		Extra:
	Exercise		**Exercise**		**Exercise**		

Exercise _____________

Set	#		#		#		Extra:
	Exercise		**Exercise**		**Exercise**		

Exercise _____________

Set	#		#		#		Extra:
	Exercise		**Exercise**		**Exercise**		

Brief notes for student

Daily Fitness Assessment

STUDENT 2

Routine Exercise Chart

Week _______________ **Date** _______________

Exercise _____________

Set	#		#		#		Extra:
	Exercise		**Exercise**		**Exercise**		

Exercise _____________

Set	#		#		#		Extra:
	Exercise		**Exercise**		**Exercise**		

Exercise _____________

Set	#		#		#		Extra:
	Exercise		**Exercise**		**Exercise**		

Exercise _____________

Set	#		#		#		Extra:
	Exercise		**Exercise**		**Exercise**		

Exercise _____________

Set	#		#		#		Extra:
	Exercise		**Exercise**		**Exercise**		

Exercise _____________

Set	#		#		#		Extra:
	Exercise		**Exercise**		**Exercise**		

Brief notes for student

Daily Fitness Assessment

STUDENT 2

Routine Exercise Chart

Week ________________ Date _______________

Exercise _____________

Set	#		#		#		Extra:
	Exercise		**Exercise**		**Exercise**		

Exercise _____________

Set	#		#		#		Extra:
	Exercise		**Exercise**		**Exercise**		

Exercise _____________

Set	#		#		#		Extra:
	Exercise		**Exercise**		**Exercise**		

Exercise _____________

Set	#		#		#		Extra:
	Exercise		**Exercise**		**Exercise**		

Exercise _____________

Set	#		#		#		Extra:
	Exercise		**Exercise**		**Exercise**		

Exercise _____________

Set	#		#		#		Extra:
	Exercise		**Exercise**		**Exercise**		

Brief notes for student

Daily Fitness Assessment

Routine Exercise Chart

Week ________________ **Date** _______________

STUDENT 2

Exercise _____________

	#	#	#	Extra:
Set	**Exercise**	**Exercise**	**Exercise**	

Exercise _____________

	#	#	#	Extra:
Set	**Exercise**	**Exercise**	**Exercise**	

Exercise _____________

	#	#	#	Extra:
Set	**Exercise**	**Exercise**	**Exercise**	

Exercise _____________

	#	#	#	Extra:
Set	**Exercise**	**Exercise**	**Exercise**	

Exercise _____________

	#	#	#	Extra:
Set	**Exercise**	**Exercise**	**Exercise**	

Exercise _____________

	#	#	#	Extra:
Set	**Exercise**	**Exercise**	**Exercise**	

Brief notes for student

Daily Fitness Assessment

Routine Exercise Chart

Week ________________ **Date** _______________

Exercise _____________

	#		#		#		Extra:
Set	**Exercise**		**Exercise**		**Exercise**		

Exercise _____________

	#		#		#		Extra:
Set	**Exercise**		**Exercise**		**Exercise**		

STUDENT 2

Exercise _____________

	#		#		#		Extra:
Set	**Exercise**		**Exercise**		**Exercise**		

Exercise _____________

	#		#		#		Extra:
Set	**Exercise**		**Exercise**		**Exercise**		

Exercise _____________

	#		#		#		Extra:
Set	**Exercise**		**Exercise**		**Exercise**		

Exercise _____________

	#		#		#		Extra:
Set	**Exercise**		**Exercise**		**Exercise**		

Brief notes for student

Daily Fitness Assessment

STUDENT 2

Routine Exercise Chart

Week ________________ **Date** _______________

Exercise _____________

Set	# Exercise	# Exercise	# Exercise	Extra:

Exercise _____________

Set	# Exercise	# Exercise	# Exercise	Extra:

Exercise _____________

Set	# Exercise	# Exercise	# Exercise	Extra:

Exercise _____________

Set	# Exercise	# Exercise	# Exercise	Extra:

Exercise _____________

Set	# Exercise	# Exercise	# Exercise	Extra:

Exercise _____________

Set	# Exercise	# Exercise	# Exercise	Extra:

Brief notes for student

Daily Fitness Assessment

STUDENT 2

Routine Exercise Chart

Week ________________ **Date** _______________

Exercise _____________

Set	# Exercise	# Exercise	# Exercise	Extra:

Exercise _____________

Set	# Exercise	# Exercise	# Exercise	Extra:

Exercise _____________

Set	# Exercise	# Exercise	# Exercise	Extra:

Exercise _____________

Set	# Exercise	# Exercise	# Exercise	Extra:

Exercise _____________

Set	# Exercise	# Exercise	# Exercise	Extra:

Exercise _____________

Set	# Exercise	# Exercise	# Exercise	Extra:

Brief notes for student

Daily Fitness Assessment

STUDENT 2

Routine Exercise Chart

Week ________________ **Date** ________________

Exercise _____________

Set	# Exercise	# Exercise	# Exercise	Extra:

Exercise _____________

Set	# Exercise	# Exercise	# Exercise	Extra:

Exercise _____________

Set	# Exercise	# Exercise	# Exercise	Extra:

Exercise _____________

Set	# Exercise	# Exercise	# Exercise	Extra:

Exercise _____________

Set	# Exercise	# Exercise	# Exercise	Extra:

Exercise _____________

Set	# Exercise	# Exercise	# Exercise	Extra:

Brief notes for student

Daily Fitness Assessment

Total Body Workout

STUDENT 2

Date ________ Date ________ Date ________

Cardio	#		#		#	
		Time		Time		Time
1. Stationary Bike						
2. Treadmill						
3. Aerobic classes						
4. Racquetball						
5. Jump rope						
6. Ski machine						
7. Jogging						
8. Jumping jacks						
9. Boxing						
10. Basketball						
11. Walking						
12. Stair stepper						
13. Swimming						
14. Volleyball						
15. Water polo						
16. Rock climbing 17. Football	Notes:		Notes:		Notes:	

Daily Fitness Assessment

STUDENT 2

Total Body Workout

	Date ________		Date ________		Date ________	
	#		#		#	
Cardio		**Time**		**Time**		**Time**
1. Stationary Bike						
2. Treadmill						
3. Aerobic classes						
4. Racquetball						
5. Jump rope						
6. Ski machine						
7. Jogging						
8. Jumping jacks						
9. Boxing						
10. Basketball						
11. Walking						
12. Stair stepper						
13. Swimming						
14. Volleyball						
15. Water polo						
16. Rock climbing	Notes:		Notes:		Notes:	
17. Football						

Daily Fitness Assessment

Total Body Workout

Date ________ **Date** ________ **Date** ________

Cardio	#		#		#	
		Time		**Time**		**Time**
1. Stationary Bike						
2. Treadmill						
3. Aerobic classes						
4. Racquetball						
5. Jump rope						
6. Ski machine						
7. Jogging						
8. Jumping jacks						
9. Boxing						
10. Basketball						
11. Walking						
12. Stair stepper						
13. Swimming						
14. Volleyball						
15. Water polo						
16. Rock climbing 17. Football	Notes:		Notes:		Notes:	

Daily Fitness Assessment

STUDENT 2

Total Body Workout

Date ________ Date ________ Date ________

Cardio	#		#		#	
		Time		Time		Time
1. Stationary Bike						
2. Treadmill						
3. Aerobic classes						
4. Racquetball						
5. Jump rope						
6. Ski machine						
7. Jogging						
8. Jumping jacks						
9. Boxing						
10. Basketball						
11. Walking						
12. Stair stepper						
13. Swimming						
14. Volleyball						
15. Water polo						
16. Rock climbing 17. Football	Notes:		Notes:		Notes:	

Daily Fitness Assessment

Total Body Workout

STUDENT 2

Date ________ **Date** ________ **Date** ________

Cardio	#		#		#	
	Time		**Time**		**Time**	
1. Stationary Bike						
2. Treadmill						
3. Aerobic classes						
4. Racquetball						
5. Jump rope						
6. Ski machine						
7. Jogging						
8. Jumping jacks						
9. Boxing						
10. Basketball						
11. Walking						
12. Stair stepper						
13. Swimming						
14. Volleyball						
15. Water polo						
16. Rock climbing	Notes:		Notes:		Notes:	
17. Football						

Student Information

Student Name ______________________________

Address ______________________________

____

Phone (cell) ______________________________

(home) ______________________________

Email ______________________________

STUDENT 3

Goals:

1.______________________
2.______________________
3.______________________
4.______________________
5.______________________
6.______________________
7.______________________
8.______________________

Body Measurements

Before		After	
Body Fat _____	Neck ______	Body Fat _____	Neck ______
Chest _____	Waist ______	Chest _____	Waist ______
Hips _____		Hips _____	
Weight _______		**Weight _______**	

Daily Fitness Assessment

Routine Exercise Chart

Week ________________ Date _______________

Exercise _____________

Set	# Exercise	# Exercise	# Exercise	Extra:

Exercise _____________

Set	# Exercise	# Exercise	# Exercise	Extra:

Exercise _____________

Set	# Exercise	# Exercise	# Exercise	Extra:

Exercise _____________

Set	# Exercise	# Exercise	# Exercise	Extra:

Exercise _____________

Set	# Exercise	# Exercise	# Exercise	Extra:

Exercise _____________

Set	# Exercise	# Exercise	# Exercise	Extra:

Brief notes for student

Daily Fitness Assessment

Routine Exercise Chart

Week ________________ **Date** _______________

Exercise _____________

Set	# Exercise	# Exercise	# Exercise	Extra:

Exercise _____________

Set	# Exercise	# Exercise	# Exercise	Extra:

Exercise _____________

Set	# Exercise	# Exercise	# Exercise	Extra:

Exercise _____________

Set	# Exercise	# Exercise	# Exercise	Extra:

Exercise _____________

Set	# Exercise	# Exercise	# Exercise	Extra:

Exercise _____________

Set	# Exercise	# Exercise	# Exercise	Extra:

Brief notes for student

Daily Fitness Assessment

Routine Exercise Chart

Week ________________ Date _______________

Exercise _____________

Set	#		#		#		Extra:
	Exercise		Exercise		Exercise		

Exercise _____________

Set	#		#		#		Extra:
	Exercise		Exercise		Exercise		

Exercise _____________

Set	#		#		#		Extra:
	Exercise		Exercise		Exercise		

Exercise _____________

Set	#		#		#		Extra:
	Exercise		Exercise		Exercise		

Exercise _____________

Set	#		#		#		Extra:
	Exercise		Exercise		Exercise		

Exercise _____________

Set	#		#		#		Extra:
	Exercise		Exercise		Exercise		

Brief notes for student

Daily Fitness Assessment

Routine Exercise Chart

Week ________________ **Date** _______________

Exercise _____________

Set	#		#		#		Extra:
	Exercise		**Exercise**		**Exercise**		

Exercise _____________

Set	#		#		#		Extra:
	Exercise		**Exercise**		**Exercise**		

Exercise _____________

Set	#		#		#		Extra:
	Exercise		**Exercise**		**Exercise**		

Exercise _____________

Set	#		#		#		Extra:
	Exercise		**Exercise**		**Exercise**		

Exercise _____________

Set	#		#		#		Extra:
	Exercise		**Exercise**		**Exercise**		

Exercise _____________

Set	#		#		#		Extra:
	Exercise		**Exercise**		**Exercise**		

Brief notes for student

Daily Fitness Assessment

Routine Exercise Chart

Week _______________ **Date** _______________

Exercise _____________

Set	#		#		#		Extra:
	Exercise		**Exercise**		**Exercise**		

Exercise _____________

Set	#		#		#		Extra:
	Exercise		**Exercise**		**Exercise**		

Exercise _____________

Set	#		#		#		Extra:
	Exercise		**Exercise**		**Exercise**		

Exercise _____________

Set	#		#		#		Extra:
	Exercise		**Exercise**		**Exercise**		

Exercise _____________

Set	#		#		#		Extra:
	Exercise		**Exercise**		**Exercise**		

Exercise _____________

Set	#		#		#		Extra:
	Exercise		**Exercise**		**Exercise**		

Brief notes for student

Daily Fitness Assessment

Routine Exercise Chart

Week ________________ **Date** ________________

Exercise ______________

Set	#		#		#		Extra:
	Exercise		**Exercise**		**Exercise**		

Exercise ______________

Set	#		#		#		Extra:
	Exercise		**Exercise**		**Exercise**		

Exercise ______________

Set	#		#		#		Extra:
	Exercise		**Exercise**		**Exercise**		

Exercise ______________

Set	#		#		#		Extra:
	Exercise		**Exercise**		**Exercise**		

Exercise ______________

Set	#		#		#		Extra:
	Exercise		**Exercise**		**Exercise**		

Exercise ______________

Set	#		#		#		Extra:
	Exercise		**Exercise**		**Exercise**		

Brief notes for student

Daily Fitness Assessment

Routine Exercise Chart

Week _______________ **Date** ______________

Exercise ____________

	#		#		#		Extra:
Set	**Exercise**		**Exercise**		**Exercise**		

Exercise ____________

	#		#		#		Extra:
Set	**Exercise**		**Exercise**		**Exercise**		

Exercise ____________

	#		#		#		Extra:
Set	**Exercise**		**Exercise**		**Exercise**		

Exercise ____________

	#		#		#		Extra:
Set	**Exercise**		**Exercise**		**Exercise**		

Exercise ____________

	#		#		#		Extra:
Set	**Exercise**		**Exercise**		**Exercise**		

Exercise ____________

	#		#		#		Extra:
Set	**Exercise**		**Exercise**		**Exercise**		

Brief notes for student

Daily Fitness Assessment

Routine Exercise Chart

Week ________________ **Date** _______________

Exercise _____________

Set	#		#		#		Extra:
	Exercise		**Exercise**		**Exercise**		

Exercise _____________

Set	#		#		#		Extra:
	Exercise		**Exercise**		**Exercise**		

Exercise _____________

Set	#		#		#		Extra:
	Exercise		**Exercise**		**Exercise**		

Exercise _____________

Set	#		#		#		Extra:
	Exercise		**Exercise**		**Exercise**		

Exercise _____________

Set	#		#		#		Extra:
	Exercise		**Exercise**		**Exercise**		

Exercise _____________

Set	#		#		#		Extra:
	Exercise		**Exercise**		**Exercise**		

Brief notes for student

Daily Fitness Assessment

Routine Exercise Chart

Week ________________ **Date** _______________

Exercise _____________

Set	# Exercise	# Exercise	# Exercise	Extra:

Exercise _____________

Set	# Exercise	# Exercise	# Exercise	Extra:

Exercise _____________

Set	# Exercise	# Exercise	# Exercise	Extra:

Exercise _____________

Set	# Exercise	# Exercise	# Exercise	Extra:

Exercise _____________

Set	# Exercise	# Exercise	# Exercise	Extra:

Exercise _____________

Set	# Exercise	# Exercise	# Exercise	Extra:

Brief notes for student

Daily Fitness Assessment

Routine Exercise Chart

Week ________________ **Date** _______________

Exercise _____________

Set	#		#		#		Extra:
	Exercise		**Exercise**		**Exercise**		

Exercise _____________

Set	#		#		#		Extra:
	Exercise		**Exercise**		**Exercise**		

Exercise _____________

Set	#		#		#		Extra:
	Exercise		**Exercise**		**Exercise**		

Exercise _____________

Set	#		#		#		Extra:
	Exercise		**Exercise**		**Exercise**		

Exercise _____________

Set	#		#		#		Extra:
	Exercise		**Exercise**		**Exercise**		

Exercise _____________

Set	#		#		#		Extra:
	Exercise		**Exercise**		**Exercise**		

Brief notes for student

Daily Fitness Assessment

Routine Exercise Chart

Week ________________ **Date** _______________

Exercise _____________

Set	#		#		#		Extra:
	Exercise		**Exercise**		**Exercise**		

Exercise _____________

Set	#		#		#		Extra:
	Exercise		**Exercise**		**Exercise**		

Exercise _____________

Set	#		#		#		Extra:
	Exercise		**Exercise**		**Exercise**		

Exercise _____________

Set	#		#		#		Extra:
	Exercise		**Exercise**		**Exercise**		

Exercise _____________

Set	#		#		#		Extra:
	Exercise		**Exercise**		**Exercise**		

Exercise _____________

Set	#		#		#		Extra:
	Exercise		**Exercise**		**Exercise**		

Brief notes for student

Daily Fitness Assessment

Routine Exercise Chart

Week ________________ **Date** ________________

Exercise ______________

Set	#		#		#		Extra:
	Exercise		**Exercise**		**Exercise**		

Exercise ______________

Set	#		#		#		Extra:
	Exercise		**Exercise**		**Exercise**		

Exercise ______________

Set	#		#		#		Extra:
	Exercise		**Exercise**		**Exercise**		

Exercise ______________

Set	#		#		#		Extra:
	Exercise		**Exercise**		**Exercise**		

Exercise ______________

Set	#		#		#		Extra:
	Exercise		**Exercise**		**Exercise**		

Exercise ______________

Set	#		#		#		Extra:
	Exercise		**Exercise**		**Exercise**		

Brief notes for student

Daily Fitness Assessment

Routine Exercise Chart

Week ________________ **Date** ________________

Exercise ______________

Set	#		#		#		Extra:
	Exercise		**Exercise**		**Exercise**		

Exercise ______________

Set	#		#		#		Extra:
	Exercise		**Exercise**		**Exercise**		

Exercise ______________

Set	#		#		#		Extra:
	Exercise		**Exercise**		**Exercise**		

Exercise ______________

Set	#		#		#		Extra:
	Exercise		**Exercise**		**Exercise**		

Exercise ______________

Set	#		#		#		Extra:
	Exercise		**Exercise**		**Exercise**		

Exercise ______________

Set	#		#		#		Extra:
	Exercise		**Exercise**		**Exercise**		

Brief notes for student

Daily Fitness Assessment

Routine Exercise Chart

Week ________________ **Date** ________________

Exercise ______________

	#	#	#	Extra:
Set	**Exercise**	**Exercise**	**Exercise**	

Exercise ______________

	#	#	#	Extra:
Set	**Exercise**	**Exercise**	**Exercise**	

Exercise ______________

	#	#	#	Extra:
Set	**Exercise**	**Exercise**	**Exercise**	

Exercise ______________

	#	#	#	Extra:
Set	**Exercise**	**Exercise**	**Exercise**	

Exercise ______________

	#	#	#	Extra:
Set	**Exercise**	**Exercise**	**Exercise**	

Exercise ______________

	#	#	#	Extra:
Set	**Exercise**	**Exercise**	**Exercise**	

Brief notes for student

Daily Fitness Assessment

Routine Exercise Chart

Week ______________ **Date** ______________

Exercise ____________

	#	#	#	Extra:
Set	**Exercise**	**Exercise**	**Exercise**	

Exercise ____________

	#	#	#	Extra:
Set	**Exercise**	**Exercise**	**Exercise**	

Exercise ____________

	#	#	#	Extra:
Set	**Exercise**	**Exercise**	**Exercise**	

Exercise ____________

	#	#	#	Extra:
Set	**Exercise**	**Exercise**	**Exercise**	

Exercise ____________

	#	#	#	Extra:
Set	**Exercise**	**Exercise**	**Exercise**	

Exercise ____________

	#	#	#	Extra:
Set	**Exercise**	**Exercise**	**Exercise**	

Brief notes for student

Daily Fitness Assessment

STUDENT 3

Total Body Workout

Cardio	Date ________		Date ________		Date ________	
	#		#		#	
		Time		Time		Time
1. Stationary Bike						
2. Treadmill						
3. Aerobic classes						
4. Racquetball						
5. Jump rope						
6. Ski machine						
7. Jogging						
8. Jumping jacks						
9. Boxing						
10. Basketball						
11. Walking						
12. Stair stepper						
13. Swimming						
14. Volleyball						
15. Water polo						
16. Rock climbing 17. Football	Notes:		Notes:		Notes:	

Daily Fitness Assessment

Total Body Workout

Date ________ Date ________ Date ________

STUDENT 3

Cardio	#		#		#	
		Time		Time		Time
1. Stationary Bike						
2. Treadmill						
3. Aerobic classes						
4. Racquetball						
5. Jump rope						
6. Ski machine						
7. Jogging						
8. Jumping jacks						
9. Boxing						
10. Basketball						
11. Walking						
12. Stair stepper						
13. Swimming						
14. Volleyball						
15. Water polo						
16. Rock climbing	Notes:		Notes:		Notes:	
17. Football						

Daily Fitness Assessment

Total Body Workout

STUDENT 3

	Date ________		Date ________		Date ________	
Cardio	#		#		#	
		Time		**Time**		**Time**
1. Stationary Bike						
2. Treadmill						
3. Aerobic classes						
4. Racquetball						
5. Jump rope						
6. Ski machine						
7. Jogging						
8. Jumping jacks						
9. Boxing						
10. Basketball						
11. Walking						
12. Stair stepper						
13. Swimming						
14. Volleyball						
15. Water polo						
16. Rock climbing	Notes:		Notes:		Notes:	
17. Football						

Daily Fitness Assessment

Total Body Workout

STUDENT 3

	Date ________		Date ________		Date ________	
	#		#		#	
Cardio		**Time**		**Time**		**Time**
1. Stationary Bike						
2. Treadmill						
3. Aerobic classes						
4. Racquetball						
5. Jump rope						
6. Ski machine						
7. Jogging						
8. Jumping jacks						
9. Boxing						
10. Basketball						
11. Walking						
12. Stair stepper						
13. Swimming						
14. Volleyball						
15. Water polo						
16. Rock climbing	Notes:		Notes:		Notes:	
17. Football						

Daily Fitness Assessment

Total Body Workout

STUDENT 3

	Date ________		Date ________		Date ________	
	#		#		#	
Cardio		**Time**		**Time**		**Time**
1. Stationary Bike						
2. Treadmill						
3. Aerobic classes						
4. Racquetball						
5. Jump rope						
6. Ski machine						
7. Jogging						
8. Jumping jacks						
9. Boxing						
10. Basketball						
11. Walking						
12. Stair stepper						
13. Swimming						
14. Volleyball						
15. Water polo						
16. Rock climbing 17. Football	Notes:		Notes:		Notes:	

Student Information

Student Name ______________________________

Address ______________________________

____

Phone (cell) ______________________________

(home) ______________________________

Email ______________________________

Goals:

1. ______________________
2. ______________________
3. ______________________
4. ______________________
5. ______________________
6. ______________________
7. ______________________
8. ______________________

STUDENT 4

Body Measurements

Before

Body Fat _____ Neck ______
Chest _____ Waist ______
Hips _____

Weight _______

After

Body Fat _____ Neck ______
Chest _____ Waist ______
Hips _____

Weight _______

Daily Fitness Assessment

Routine Exercise Chart

Week ________________ **Date** _______________

Exercise _____________

Set	#		#		#		Extra:
	Exercise		**Exercise**		**Exercise**		

Exercise _____________

Set	#		#		#		Extra:
	Exercise		**Exercise**		**Exercise**		

Exercise _____________

Set	#		#		#		Extra:
	Exercise		**Exercise**		**Exercise**		

Exercise _____________

Set	#		#		#		Extra:
	Exercise		**Exercise**		**Exercise**		

Exercise _____________

Set	#		#		#		Extra:
	Exercise		**Exercise**		**Exercise**		

Exercise _____________

Set	#		#		#		Extra:
	Exercise		**Exercise**		**Exercise**		

Brief notes for student

Daily Fitness Assessment

Routine Exercise Chart

Week ______________ **Date** ______________

Exercise ____________

Set	#		#		#		Extra:
	Exercise		**Exercise**		**Exercise**		

Exercise ____________

Set	#		#		#		Extra:
	Exercise		**Exercise**		**Exercise**		

Exercise ____________

Set	#		#		#		Extra:
	Exercise		**Exercise**		**Exercise**		

Exercise ____________

Set	#		#		#		Extra:
	Exercise		**Exercise**		**Exercise**		

Exercise ____________

Set	#		#		#		Extra:
	Exercise		**Exercise**		**Exercise**		

Exercise ____________

Set	#		#		#		Extra:
	Exercise		**Exercise**		**Exercise**		

Brief notes for student

Daily Fitness Assessment

Routine Exercise Chart

Week _______________ **Date** _______________

Exercise _____________

	#	#	#	Extra:
Set	**Exercise**	**Exercise**	**Exercise**	

Exercise _____________

	#	#	#	Extra:
Set	**Exercise**	**Exercise**	**Exercise**	

Exercise _____________

	#	#	#	Extra:
Set	**Exercise**	**Exercise**	**Exercise**	

Exercise _____________

	#	#	#	Extra:
Set	**Exercise**	**Exercise**	**Exercise**	

Exercise _____________

	#	#	#	Extra:
Set	**Exercise**	**Exercise**	**Exercise**	

Exercise _____________

	#	#	#	Extra:
Set	**Exercise**	**Exercise**	**Exercise**	

Brief notes for student

Daily Fitness Assessment

Routine Exercise Chart

Week ______________ **Date** ______________

Exercise ____________

	#	#	#	Extra:
Set	**Exercise**	**Exercise**	**Exercise**	

Exercise ____________

	#	#	#	Extra:
Set	**Exercise**	**Exercise**	**Exercise**	

Exercise ____________

	#	#	#	Extra:
Set	**Exercise**	**Exercise**	**Exercise**	

Exercise ____________

	#	#	#	Extra:
Set	**Exercise**	**Exercise**	**Exercise**	

Exercise ____________

	#	#	#	Extra:
Set	**Exercise**	**Exercise**	**Exercise**	

Exercise ____________

	#	#	#	Extra:
Set	**Exercise**	**Exercise**	**Exercise**	

Brief notes for student

Daily Fitness Assessment

Routine Exercise Chart

Week ________________ Date ________________

Exercise ______________

Set	#	#	#	Extra:
	Exercise	**Exercise**	**Exercise**	

Exercise ______________

Set	#	#	#	Extra:
	Exercise	**Exercise**	**Exercise**	

Exercise ______________

Set	#	#	#	Extra:
	Exercise	**Exercise**	**Exercise**	

Exercise ______________

Set	#	#	#	Extra:
	Exercise	**Exercise**	**Exercise**	

Exercise ______________

Set	#	#	#	Extra:
	Exercise	**Exercise**	**Exercise**	

Exercise ______________

Set	#	#	#	Extra:
	Exercise	**Exercise**	**Exercise**	

Brief notes for student

Daily Fitness Assessment

Routine Exercise Chart

Week ________________ **Date** _______________

Exercise _____________

	#	#	#	Extra:
Set	**Exercise**	**Exercise**	**Exercise**	

Exercise _____________

	#	#	#	Extra:
Set	**Exercise**	**Exercise**	**Exercise**	

Exercise _____________

	#	#	#	Extra:
Set	**Exercise**	**Exercise**	**Exercise**	

Exercise _____________

	#	#	#	Extra:
Set	**Exercise**	**Exercise**	**Exercise**	

Exercise _____________

	#	#	#	Extra:
Set	**Exercise**	**Exercise**	**Exercise**	

Exercise _____________

	#	#	#	Extra:
Set	**Exercise**	**Exercise**	**Exercise**	

Brief notes for student

Daily Fitness Assessment

Routine Exercise Chart

Week _______________ **Date** ______________

Exercise ____________

Set	#		#		#		Extra:
	Exercise		**Exercise**		**Exercise**		

Exercise ____________

Set	#		#		#		Extra:
	Exercise		**Exercise**		**Exercise**		

Exercise ____________

Set	#		#		#		Extra:
	Exercise		**Exercise**		**Exercise**		

Exercise ____________

Set	#		#		#		Extra:
	Exercise		**Exercise**		**Exercise**		

Exercise ____________

Set	#		#		#		Extra:
	Exercise		**Exercise**		**Exercise**		

Exercise ____________

Set	#		#		#		Extra:
	Exercise		**Exercise**		**Exercise**		

Brief notes for student

Daily Fitness Assessment

Routine Exercise Chart

Week _______________ **Date** _______________

Exercise _____________

Set	#		#		#		Extra:
	Exercise		**Exercise**		**Exercise**		

Exercise _____________

Set	#		#		#		Extra:
	Exercise		**Exercise**		**Exercise**		

Exercise _____________

Set	#		#		#		Extra:
	Exercise		**Exercise**		**Exercise**		

Exercise _____________

Set	#		#		#		Extra:
	Exercise		**Exercise**		**Exercise**		

Exercise _____________

Set	#		#		#		Extra:
	Exercise		**Exercise**		**Exercise**		

Exercise _____________

Set	#		#		#		Extra:
	Exercise		**Exercise**		**Exercise**		

Brief notes for student

Daily Fitness Assessment

Routine Exercise Chart

Week ________________ **Date** _______________

Exercise _____________

Set	#		#		#		Extra:
	Exercise		**Exercise**		**Exercise**		

Exercise _____________

Set	#		#		#		Extra:
	Exercise		**Exercise**		**Exercise**		

Exercise _____________

Set	#		#		#		Extra:
	Exercise		**Exercise**		**Exercise**		

Exercise _____________

Set	#		#		#		Extra:
	Exercise		**Exercise**		**Exercise**		

Exercise _____________

Set	#		#		#		Extra:
	Exercise		**Exercise**		**Exercise**		

Exercise _____________

Set	#		#		#		Extra:
	Exercise		**Exercise**		**Exercise**		

Brief notes for student

Daily Fitness Assessment

Routine Exercise Chart

Week ________________ **Date** _______________

Exercise _____________

	#	#	#	Extra:
Set	**Exercise**	**Exercise**	**Exercise**	

Exercise _____________

	#	#	#	Extra:
Set	**Exercise**	**Exercise**	**Exercise**	

Exercise _____________

	#	#	#	Extra:
Set	**Exercise**	**Exercise**	**Exercise**	

Exercise _____________

	#	#	#	Extra:
Set	**Exercise**	**Exercise**	**Exercise**	

Exercise _____________

	#	#	#	Extra:
Set	**Exercise**	**Exercise**	**Exercise**	

Exercise _____________

	#	#	#	Extra:
Set	**Exercise**	**Exercise**	**Exercise**	

Brief notes for student

Daily Fitness Assessment

Routine Exercise Chart

Week ________________ **Date** _______________

Exercise _____________

Set	#		#		#		Extra:
	Exercise		**Exercise**		**Exercise**		

Exercise _____________

Set	#		#		#		Extra:
	Exercise		**Exercise**		**Exercise**		

Exercise _____________

Set	#		#		#		Extra:
	Exercise		**Exercise**		**Exercise**		

Exercise _____________

Set	#		#		#		Extra:
	Exercise		**Exercise**		**Exercise**		

Exercise _____________

Set	#		#		#		Extra:
	Exercise		**Exercise**		**Exercise**		

Exercise _____________

Set	#		#		#		Extra:
	Exercise		**Exercise**		**Exercise**		

Brief notes for student

Daily Fitness Assessment

Routine Exercise Chart

Week _______________ **Date** _______________

Exercise _____________

Set	#		#		#		Extra:
	Exercise		**Exercise**		**Exercise**		

Exercise _____________

Set	#		#		#		Extra:
	Exercise		**Exercise**		**Exercise**		

Exercise _____________

Set	#		#		#		Extra:
	Exercise		**Exercise**		**Exercise**		

Exercise _____________

Set	#		#		#		Extra:
	Exercise		**Exercise**		**Exercise**		

Exercise _____________

Set	#		#		#		Extra:
	Exercise		**Exercise**		**Exercise**		

Exercise _____________

Set	#		#		#		Extra:
	Exercise		**Exercise**		**Exercise**		

Brief notes for student

Daily Fitness Assessment

Routine Exercise Chart

Week ________________ **Date** ________________

Exercise ______________

Set	#		#		#		Extra:
	Exercise		**Exercise**		**Exercise**		

Exercise ______________

Set	#		#		#		Extra:
	Exercise		**Exercise**		**Exercise**		

Exercise ______________

Set	#		#		#		Extra:
	Exercise		**Exercise**		**Exercise**		

Exercise ______________

Set	#		#		#		Extra:
	Exercise		**Exercise**		**Exercise**		

Exercise ______________

Set	#		#		#		Extra:
	Exercise		**Exercise**		**Exercise**		

Exercise ______________

Set	#		#		#		Extra:
	Exercise		**Exercise**		**Exercise**		

Brief notes for student

Daily Fitness Assessment

Routine Exercise Chart

Week ________________ **Date** _______________

Exercise _____________

Set	# Exercise	# Exercise	# Exercise	Extra:

Exercise _____________

Set	# Exercise	# Exercise	# Exercise	Extra:

Exercise _____________

Set	# Exercise	# Exercise	# Exercise	Extra:

Exercise _____________

Set	# Exercise	# Exercise	# Exercise	Extra:

Exercise _____________

Set	# Exercise	# Exercise	# Exercise	Extra:

Exercise _____________

Set	# Exercise	# Exercise	# Exercise	Extra:

Brief notes for student

Daily Fitness Assessment

Routine Exercise Chart

Week ______________ **Date** ______________

Exercise ____________

Set	#		#		#		Extra:
	Exercise		**Exercise**		**Exercise**		

Exercise ____________

Set	#		#		#		Extra:
	Exercise		**Exercise**		**Exercise**		

Exercise ____________

Set	#		#		#		Extra:
	Exercise		**Exercise**		**Exercise**		

Exercise ____________

Set	#		#		#		Extra:
	Exercise		**Exercise**		**Exercise**		

Exercise ____________

Set	#		#		#		Extra:
	Exercise		**Exercise**		**Exercise**		

Exercise ____________

Set	#		#		#		Extra:
	Exercise		**Exercise**		**Exercise**		

Brief notes for student

Daily Fitness Assessment

Total Body Workout

	Date ________		Date ________		Date ________	
	#		#		#	
Cardio		**Time**		**Time**		**Time**
1. Stationary Bike						
2. Treadmill						
3. Aerobic classes						
4. Racquetball						
5. Jump rope						
6. Ski machine						
7. Jogging						
8. Jumping jacks						
9. Boxing						
10. Basketball						
11. Walking						
12. Stair stepper						
13. Swimming						
14. Volleyball						
15. Water polo						
16. Rock climbing	Notes:		Notes:		Notes:	
17. Football						

STUDENT 4

Daily Fitness Assessment

Total Body Workout

	Date ________		Date ________		Date ________	
	#		#		#	
Cardio		**Time**		**Time**		**Time**
1. Stationary Bike						
2. Treadmill						
3. Aerobic classes						
4. Racquetball						
5. Jump rope						
6. Ski machine						
7. Jogging						
8. Jumping jacks						
9. Boxing						
10. Basketball						
11. Walking						
12. Stair stepper						
13. Swimming						
14. Volleyball						
15. Water polo						
16. Rock climbing	Notes:		Notes:		Notes:	
17. Football						

STUDENT 4

Daily Fitness Assessment

Total Body Workout

Cardio	Date ________		Date ________		Date ________	
	#		#		#	
		Time		Time		Time
1. Stationary Bike						
2. Treadmill						
3. Aerobic classes						
4. Racquetball						
5. Jump rope						
6. Ski machine						
7. Jogging						
8. Jumping jacks						
9. Boxing						
10. Basketball						
11. Walking						
12. Stair stepper						
13. Swimming						
14. Volleyball						
15. Water polo						
16. Rock climbing	Notes:		Notes:		Notes:	
17. Football						

STUDENT 4

Daily Fitness Assessment

Total Body Workout

	Date ________		Date ________		Date ________	
Cardio	#	Time	#	Time	#	Time
1. Stationary Bike						
2. Treadmill						
3. Aerobic classes						
4. Racquetball						
5. Jump rope						
6. Ski machine						
7. Jogging						
8. Jumping jacks						
9. Boxing						
10. Basketball						
11. Walking						
12. Stair stepper						
13. Swimming						
14. Volleyball						
15. Water polo						
16. Rock climbing	Notes:		Notes:		Notes:	
17. Football						

STUDENT 4

Daily Fitness Assessment

Total Body Workout

Date ________ **Date** ________ **Date** ________

Cardio	#		#		#	
		Time		**Time**		**Time**
1. Stationary Bike						
2. Treadmill						
3. Aerobic classes						
4. Racquetball						
5. Jump rope						
6. Ski machine						
7. Jogging						
8. Jumping jacks						
9. Boxing						
10. Basketball						
11. Walking						
12. Stair stepper						
13. Swimming						
14. Volleyball						
15. Water polo						
16. Rock climbing 17. Football	Notes:		Notes:		Notes:	

STUDENT 4

Student Information

Student Name ______________________________

Address ______________________________

____

Phone (cell) ______________________________

(home) ______________________________

Email ______________________________

Goals:

1. ______________________
2. ______________________
3. ______________________
4. ______________________
5. ______________________
6. ______________________
7. ______________________
8. ______________________

STUDENT 5

Body Measurements

Before

Body Fat _____ Neck ______
Chest _____ Waist ______
Hips _____

Weight _______

After

Body Fat _____ Neck ______
Chest _____ Waist ______
Hips _____

Weight _______

Daily Fitness Assessment

Routine Exercise Chart

Week ________________ Date _______________

Exercise _____________

Set	# Exercise	# Exercise	# Exercise	Extra:

Exercise _____________

Set	# Exercise	# Exercise	# Exercise	Extra:

Exercise _____________

Set	# Exercise	# Exercise	# Exercise	Extra:

Exercise _____________

Set	# Exercise	# Exercise	# Exercise	Extra:

Exercise _____________

Set	# Exercise	# Exercise	# Exercise	Extra:

Exercise _____________

Set	# Exercise	# Exercise	# Exercise	Extra:

Brief notes for student

Daily Fitness Assessment

Routine Exercise Chart

Week ______________ Date ______________

Exercise ____________

Set	#		#		#		Extra:
	Exercise		**Exercise**		**Exercise**		

Exercise ____________

Set	#		#		#		Extra:
	Exercise		**Exercise**		**Exercise**		

Exercise ____________

Set	#		#		#		Extra:
	Exercise		**Exercise**		**Exercise**		

Exercise ____________

Set	#		#		#		Extra:
	Exercise		**Exercise**		**Exercise**		

Exercise ____________

Set	#		#		#		Extra:
	Exercise		**Exercise**		**Exercise**		

Exercise ____________

Set	#		#		#		Extra:
	Exercise		**Exercise**		**Exercise**		

Brief notes for student

Daily Fitness Assessment

Routine Exercise Chart

Week ________________ **Date** _______________

Exercise _____________

Set	#		#		#		Extra:
	Exercise		**Exercise**		**Exercise**		

Exercise _____________

Set	#		#		#		Extra:
	Exercise		**Exercise**		**Exercise**		

Exercise _____________

Set	#		#		#		Extra:
	Exercise		**Exercise**		**Exercise**		

Exercise _____________

Set	#		#		#		Extra:
	Exercise		**Exercise**		**Exercise**		

Exercise _____________

Set	#		#		#		Extra:
	Exercise		**Exercise**		**Exercise**		

Exercise _____________

Set	#		#		#		Extra:
	Exercise		**Exercise**		**Exercise**		

Brief notes for student

Daily Fitness Assessment

Routine Exercise Chart

Week ________________ **Date** _______________

Exercise _____________

Set	#		#		#		Extra:
	Exercise		**Exercise**		**Exercise**		

Exercise _____________

Set	#		#		#		Extra:
	Exercise		**Exercise**		**Exercise**		

Exercise _____________

Set	#		#		#		Extra:
	Exercise		**Exercise**		**Exercise**		

Exercise _____________

Set	#		#		#		Extra:
	Exercise		**Exercise**		**Exercise**		

Exercise _____________

Set	#		#		#		Extra:
	Exercise		**Exercise**		**Exercise**		

Exercise _____________

Set	#		#		#		Extra:
	Exercise		**Exercise**		**Exercise**		

Brief notes for student

Daily Fitness Assessment

Routine Exercise Chart

Week ________________ **Date** ______________

Exercise _____________

Set	#	#	#	Extra:
	Exercise	**Exercise**	**Exercise**	

Exercise _____________

Set	#	#	#	Extra:
	Exercise	**Exercise**	**Exercise**	

Exercise _____________

Set	#	#	#	Extra:
	Exercise	**Exercise**	**Exercise**	

Exercise _____________

Set	#	#	#	Extra:
	Exercise	**Exercise**	**Exercise**	

Exercise _____________

Set	#	#	#	Extra:
	Exercise	**Exercise**	**Exercise**	

Exercise _____________

Set	#	#	#	Extra:
	Exercise	**Exercise**	**Exercise**	

Brief notes for student

Daily Fitness Assessment

Routine Exercise Chart

Week ________________ Date ________________

Exercise ______________

Set	#		#		#		Extra:
	Exercise		**Exercise**		**Exercise**		

Exercise ______________

Set	#		#		#		Extra:
	Exercise		**Exercise**		**Exercise**		

Exercise ______________

Set	#		#		#		Extra:
	Exercise		**Exercise**		**Exercise**		

Exercise ______________

Set	#		#		#		Extra:
	Exercise		**Exercise**		**Exercise**		

Exercise ______________

Set	#		#		#		Extra:
	Exercise		**Exercise**		**Exercise**		

Exercise ______________

Set	#		#		#		Extra:
	Exercise		**Exercise**		**Exercise**		

Brief notes for student

Daily Fitness Assessment

Routine Exercise Chart

Week _______________ Date _______________

Exercise _____________

Set	#	#	#	Extra:
	Exercise	**Exercise**	**Exercise**	

Exercise _____________

Set	#	#	#	Extra:
	Exercise	**Exercise**	**Exercise**	

Exercise _____________

Set	#	#	#	Extra:
	Exercise	**Exercise**	**Exercise**	

Exercise _____________

Set	#	#	#	Extra:
	Exercise	**Exercise**	**Exercise**	

Exercise _____________

Set	#	#	#	Extra:
	Exercise	**Exercise**	**Exercise**	

Exercise _____________

Set	#	#	#	Extra:
	Exercise	**Exercise**	**Exercise**	

Brief notes for student

Daily Fitness Assessment

Routine Exercise Chart

Week ______________ Date ______________

Exercise ____________

Set	#		#		#		Extra:
	Exercise		Exercise		Exercise		

Exercise ____________

Set	#		#		#		Extra:
	Exercise		Exercise		Exercise		

Exercise ____________

Set	#		#		#		Extra:
	Exercise		Exercise		Exercise		

Exercise ____________

Set	#		#		#		Extra:
	Exercise		Exercise		Exercise		

Exercise ____________

Set	#		#		#		Extra:
	Exercise		Exercise		Exercise		

Exercise ____________

Set	#		#		#		Extra:
	Exercise		Exercise		Exercise		

Brief notes for student

Daily Fitness Assessment

Routine Exercise Chart

Week ________________ **Date** ________________

Exercise ____________

Set	#		#		#		Extra:
	Exercise		**Exercise**		**Exercise**		

Exercise ____________

Set	#		#		#		Extra:
	Exercise		**Exercise**		**Exercise**		

Exercise ____________

Set	#		#		#		Extra:
	Exercise		**Exercise**		**Exercise**		

Exercise ____________

Set	#		#		#		Extra:
	Exercise		**Exercise**		**Exercise**		

Exercise ____________

Set	#		#		#		Extra:
	Exercise		**Exercise**		**Exercise**		

Exercise ____________

Set	#		#		#		Extra:
	Exercise		**Exercise**		**Exercise**		

Brief notes for student

Daily Fitness Assessment

Routine Exercise Chart

Week ________________ **Date** ______________

Exercise _____________

Set	#		#		#		Extra:
	Exercise		**Exercise**		**Exercise**		

Exercise _____________

Set	#		#		#		Extra:
	Exercise		**Exercise**		**Exercise**		

Exercise _____________

Set	#		#		#		Extra:
	Exercise		**Exercise**		**Exercise**		

Exercise _____________

Set	#		#		#		Extra:
	Exercise		**Exercise**		**Exercise**		

Exercise _____________

Set	#		#		#		Extra:
	Exercise		**Exercise**		**Exercise**		

Exercise _____________

Set	#		#		#		Extra:
	Exercise		**Exercise**		**Exercise**		

Brief notes for student

Daily Fitness Assessment

Routine Exercise Chart

Week ________________ **Date** _______________

Exercise _____________

	#	#	#	Extra:
Set	**Exercise**	**Exercise**	**Exercise**	

Exercise _____________

	#	#	#	Extra:
Set	**Exercise**	**Exercise**	**Exercise**	

Exercise _____________

	#	#	#	Extra:
Set	**Exercise**	**Exercise**	**Exercise**	

Exercise _____________

	#	#	#	Extra:
Set	**Exercise**	**Exercise**	**Exercise**	

Exercise _____________

	#	#	#	Extra:
Set	**Exercise**	**Exercise**	**Exercise**	

Exercise _____________

	#	#	#	Extra:
Set	**Exercise**	**Exercise**	**Exercise**	

Brief notes for student

Daily Fitness Assessment

Routine Exercise Chart

Week ________________ **Date** _______________

Exercise _____________

Set	#		#		#		Extra:
	Exercise		**Exercise**		**Exercise**		

Exercise _____________

Set	#		#		#		Extra:
	Exercise		**Exercise**		**Exercise**		

Exercise _____________

Set	#		#		#		Extra:
	Exercise		**Exercise**		**Exercise**		

Exercise _____________

Set	#		#		#		Extra:
	Exercise		**Exercise**		**Exercise**		

Exercise _____________

Set	#		#		#		Extra:
	Exercise		**Exercise**		**Exercise**		

Exercise _____________

Set	#		#		#		Extra:
	Exercise		**Exercise**		**Exercise**		

Brief notes for student

Daily Fitness Assessment

Routine Exercise Chart

Week ________________ **Date** _______________

Exercise _____________

Set	#		#		#		Extra:
	Exercise		**Exercise**		**Exercise**		

Exercise _____________

Set	#		#		#		Extra:
	Exercise		**Exercise**		**Exercise**		

Exercise _____________

Set	#		#		#		Extra:
	Exercise		**Exercise**		**Exercise**		

Exercise _____________

Set	#		#		#		Extra:
	Exercise		**Exercise**		**Exercise**		

Exercise _____________

Set	#		#		#		Extra:
	Exercise		**Exercise**		**Exercise**		

Exercise _____________

Set	#		#		#		Extra:
	Exercise		**Exercise**		**Exercise**		

Brief notes for student

Daily Fitness Assessment

Routine Exercise Chart

Week ________________ **Date** _______________

Exercise _____________

Set	#		#		#		Extra:
	Exercise		**Exercise**		**Exercise**		

Exercise _____________

Set	#		#		#		Extra:
	Exercise		**Exercise**		**Exercise**		

Exercise _____________

Set	#		#		#		Extra:
	Exercise		**Exercise**		**Exercise**		

Exercise _____________

Set	#		#		#		Extra:
	Exercise		**Exercise**		**Exercise**		

Exercise _____________

Set	#		#		#		Extra:
	Exercise		**Exercise**		**Exercise**		

Exercise _____________

Set	#		#		#		Extra:
	Exercise		**Exercise**		**Exercise**		

Brief notes for student

Daily Fitness Assessment

Routine Exercise Chart

Week ________________ **Date** ________________

Exercise ______________

Set	#		#		#		Extra:
	Exercise		**Exercise**		**Exercise**		

Exercise ______________

Set	#		#		#		Extra:
	Exercise		**Exercise**		**Exercise**		

Exercise ______________

Set	#		#		#		Extra:
	Exercise		**Exercise**		**Exercise**		

Exercise ______________

Set	#		#		#		Extra:
	Exercise		**Exercise**		**Exercise**		

Exercise ______________

Set	#		#		#		Extra:
	Exercise		**Exercise**		**Exercise**		

Exercise ______________

Set	#		#		#		Extra:
	Exercise		**Exercise**		**Exercise**		

Brief notes for student

Daily Fitness Assessment

Total Body Workout

	Date ________		Date ________		Date ________	
	#		#		#	
Cardio		**Time**		**Time**		**Time**
1. Stationary Bike						
2. Treadmill						
3. Aerobic classes						
4. Racquetball						
5. Jump rope						
6. Ski machine						
7. Jogging						
8. Jumping jacks						
9. Boxing						
10. Basketball						
11. Walking						
12. Stair stepper						
13. Swimming						
14. Volleyball						
15. Water polo						
16. Rock climbing	Notes:		Notes:		Notes:	
17. Football						

Daily Fitness Assessment

Total Body Workout

	Date ________		Date ________		Date ________	
Cardio	#	**Time**	#	**Time**	#	**Time**
1. Stationary Bike						
2. Treadmill						
3. Aerobic classes						
4. Racquetball						
5. Jump rope						
6. Ski machine						
7. Jogging						
8. Jumping jacks						
9. Boxing						
10. Basketball						
11. Walking						
12. Stair stepper						
13. Swimming						
14. Volleyball						
15. Water polo						
16. Rock climbing	Notes:		Notes:		Notes:	
17. Football						

Daily Fitness Assessment

Total Body Workout

	Date ________		Date ________		Date ________	
	#		#		#	
Cardio		**Time**		**Time**		**Time**
1. Stationary Bike						
2. Treadmill						
3. Aerobic classes						
4. Racquetball						
5. Jump rope						
6. Ski machine						
7. Jogging						
8. Jumping jacks						
9. Boxing						
10. Basketball						
11. Walking						
12. Stair stepper						
13. Swimming						
14. Volleyball						
15. Water polo						
16. Rock climbing	Notes:		Notes:		Notes:	
17. Football						

STUDENT 5

Daily Fitness Assessment

Total Body Workout

Date ________ Date ________ Date ________

Cardio	#		#		#	
		Time		Time		Time
1. Stationary Bike						
2. Treadmill						
3. Aerobic classes						
4. Racquetball						
5. Jump rope						
6. Ski machine						
7. Jogging						
8. Jumping jacks						
9. Boxing						
10. Basketball						
11. Walking						
12. Stair stepper						
13. Swimming						
14. Volleyball						
15. Water polo						
16. Rock climbing	Notes:		Notes:		Notes:	
17. Football						

Daily Fitness Assessment

Total Body Workout

Date ________ Date ________ Date ________

Cardio	#	Time	#	Time	#	Time
1. Stationary Bike						
2. Treadmill						
3. Aerobic classes						
4. Racquetball						
5. Jump rope						
6. Ski machine						
7. Jogging						
8. Jumping jacks						
9. Boxing						
10. Basketball						
11. Walking						
12. Stair stepper						
13. Swimming						
14. Volleyball						
15. Water polo						
16. Rock climbing	Notes:		Notes:		Notes:	
17. Football						

www.ingramcontent.com/pod-product-compliance
Lightning Source LLC
Chambersburg PA
CBHW051956280526
45793CB00005B/736

* 9 7 8 1 4 2 5 9 2 4 3 8 6 *